The Impending Death of Hospitals: Why You Must Plan Your Medical Practice's Survival

MARK F. WEISS

Published by Kidiakedes Omnimedia

For information about Mark F. Weiss's services and speaking, please call 310-843-2800 or email request@advisorylawgroup.com. Free articles, videos, podcasts and the archive of the Advisory e-Alert, our electronic newsletter, are available at www.advisorylawgroup.com. The Mark F. Weiss Law Firm, a Professional Corporation, 1227 De La Vina Street, Santa Barbara, CA 93101

Visit www.advisorylawgroup.com to subscribe to our complimentary monthly e-Alert and to follow the link to Mark's frequently updated Wisdom. Applied. blog.

Contents

INTRODUCTION

Hospitals have fallen for a fallacy. Now it's going to kill them. Having fallen for the fallacy that there's profit in market share, hospitals have gorged on acquisitions and on employment and alignment of physicians.

Many physicians have been willing participants through practice sales and in the belief that there's safety in hospital employment.

But it's becoming evident that physician employment leads to losses and that integrated care delivers neither better care nor lower costs.

And now, technology is about to moot many of the reasons for a hospital's existence.

How can your practice survive and even thrive in the post-hospital world? On the pages that follow, you'll learn why hospitals have become more fragile as a result of their fattening, how technological advances will gut them of many of their current functions, and what you must begin doing to assure your survival and success.

Chapter 1
CRYSTAL BALL

There are those who can see and benefit from the future. How would you like to know exactly what's going to happen in the future such that by doing so, you're going to be able to know how both to prepare for it and to profit from it?

The NHL great, Wayne Gretzky spoke about skating to where the puck is going to be. He's perhaps the only hockey player to have had that ability. The game is very complicated.

But the healthcare business is infinitely more complicated because there's not just one puck in the game, there are many. And, the barrier to entry is relatively low, and becoming lower, enabling someone to toss in a new puck and another and another.

The pucks in healthcare are, of course, are trends. Trends that are as clear as can be, if you are paying attention to them. A piece here. A piece there.

Most ignore the trends because they are blinded by the everyday. But the problem with spotting trends is that they tend to be overlooked as we go about our daily lives. Some physicians might complain that they are too busy treating patients to pay attention to trends. But how's that working out for you? Hospitals control a huge percentage of physician practices. Large national and regional companies control another swath of what used to be physician-owned practices.

Trends themselves are nothing new. They are an inherent part of business life and of our economic system.

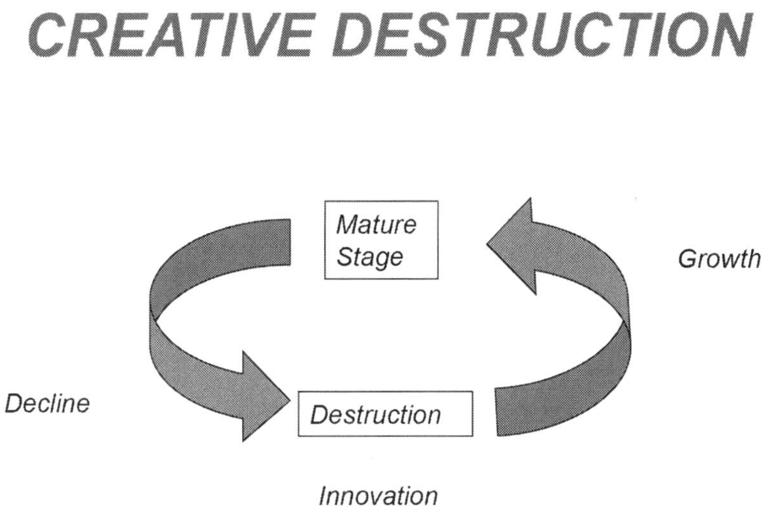

Creative destruction. The economist Joseph Schumpeter wrote in *Capitalism, Socialism and Democracy* that capitalism "is by nature a form or method of economic change and not only never is, but never can be, stationary.

And this evolutionary character … incessantly revolutionizes the economic structure from within, incessantly destroying the old one, incessantly creating a new one. This process of Creative Destruction is the essential fact about capitalism."

Trends are the footprints in the sand on the beach of economic change. Sure, trends may be fleeting and easily erased. But something made those prints, and that something is often not as ephemeral.

In this short book, we're going to review some of the trends currently impacting, and soon to impact, healthcare.
There is absolutely no question that they are going to have an impact on your business.

There is absolutely no question that they are going to have an impact on the future of hospitals.

In fact, my premise is that these trends will lead to the destruction of hospitals as we know them.

Some are fearful of these changes, perhaps of any change. They want change to stop. In fact, some take affirmative action to stop it: They lobby. They pass laws. They adopt regulations. They make economic threats.

But in the grand scheme, those efforts won't amount to anything.

For no matter what, change is inevitable.

Others run toward change. Others, and I sincerely hope that you're among them, realize that they must change their business model to take advantage of the opportunity that awaits in the direction that things are headed. They're skating toward where the puck will be, not running from it before they're hit.

Chapter 2
THE "PAST" OF HOSPITALS

To appreciate the future of hospitals, we need to take a look at their past. Our investigation of the future of healthcare centers around the future, or, as we shall see, the lack thereof, of hospitals. That's because, as we'll discuss, healthcare has become centered around hospitals. But it wasn't always that way.

The history of hospitals themselves goes back thousands of years, as far back as the Greeks and ancient Chinese.

In the Western tradition, there was initially a close tie between religious orders and charity care for the ill, which still exists today.

In the United States, the first public hospital was formed in Philadelphia in 1751 by Benjamin Franklin and Dr. Thomas Bond.

Those who could afford medical care received it from physicians at home.

But what of the poor? That's what Franklin and Bond asked.

Hospital as substitute for home-based care. The hospital envisioned by Franklin and Bond was the means of providing medical care to patients who either had no homes or who were poor and could not otherwise afford care.

This notion of caring for the public continued with the growth of religious charted institutions. Again, those who could afford care did so privately.

Physicians often pressed for the creation of publicly-owned, that is, community, hospitals, and physicians began to build clinics, that is hospitals, as an extension of their practices.

In other words, hospitals were adjunct to medical practice. Medical practice was not adjunct to hospitals.

Then hospitals bulked up. But over the many years, decades, and centuries that followed, hospitals became larger and larger in order to meet the needs of patients.

The technology of the various times made it more efficient to centralize equipment and the attendant care of patients. It also made it more efficient to provide centralized observation and monitoring. If a patient was going to be watched, what better place, they posited, than the hospital?

Medical practice vs. hospital. And yet, throughout those hundreds of years there was still a clear line between the practice of medicine and the hospital itself.

Of course, large hospitals and chains, beginning with the more or less failed attempts to bind physicians to fealty as a result of managed care in the 1980s, developed employed staffs and related medical foundations or more of less captive medical groups.

But with the near total collapse of the staff-based model in the 1990s, many hospitals withdrew from the unprofitable business of attempting to control physicians.

But note that even then, HIPAA itself was predicated on the sharing, ***the portability***, of health information across independent practitioners. Not the hoarding of information within the EMR silos of separate hospitals.

Chapter 3
GOVERNMENT INDUCES PHYSICIAN LABOR

Then, of course, along came Obamacare. The government chooses sides: Crony capitalism. Obamacare favors the growth of hospitals with its incentives for aligning physicians and hospitals.

Think ACOs and other incentives to coordinate care, meaning coordination via hospitals.

Although reports lag by several years, at least 20% to 30% of all practicing physicians are currently employed by hospitals. We do know that there was a 34 % increase in hospital employment of physicians between 2000 and 2010.

In addition, there's an uncertain number of physicians, a likely significant number, who are controlled by hospitals through alignment relationships such as ACOs and foundation model medical groups.

In fact, in some specialties the numbers are even higher. For example, it's been estimated that up to 60% of cardiologists are hospital-employed.

There are factors other than Obamacare stoking the fire. For example hospitals receive higher fees from Medicare, and often from private payors, for their employed physicians' services than those physicians received or would have received had they been in private practice.

A New York Times article by Margot Sanger-Katz cites the huge discrepancy in Medicare reimbursement for a cardiac ultrasound performed in a physician's private practice office ($189) compared with the same service by that same physician in the same office after the practice is purchased by the local hospital ($453).

And, in keeping with a fact that has remained the same ever since hospitals came into existence, other than patients entering via the ER, patients are referred to a hospital by *physicians.* Certainly, internal medicine and other primary care physicians yield a huge amount of weight here, but so do specialists and their decision about where to perform a procedure. So hospital employment and other tight alignment such as ACOs serve to bind physicians' loyalty to the facility.

Chapter 4
HOSPITAL MERGER MANIA

Cannibalism. As hospitals gobbled up physician practices, hospitals began gobbling each other up as well.

In 2013 there were 105 hospital mergers. In 2014 there were a few less, approximately 100. Overall, since 2010, there has been a 44% increase in the number of mergers.

Value-Based Purchasing. Perhaps the greatest driver is the fact that payment is transitioning from fee for service to performance and outcomes-based models. That is, to so called value-based models. Hospitals fear that this will result in lowered payments (it will) and believe that merging reduces the cost of delivery due to economies of scale.

General financial pressure is a driver. Additionally, general financial pressure is a key driver of hospital mergers. This is a very important factor that many ignore even though it's highly publicized. In fact, it's one of the most significant drivers that will result in the death of hospitals as we know them.

Hospitals merge because they think there's strength in a larger entity. If that means that two hospitals merge and become one and one facility closes down, perhaps that's the case. But that's not the general trend. Instead mergers are used to build bigger hospital systems.

But with declining occupancy rates and the resulting fewer dollars, will large hospitals and especially large hospital systems be able to stay afloat?

Doomed to ignore history. In the 1990s, a similar wave of hospital mergers led to many hospital failures. In fact, most merged hospitals failed. The same argument about economies of sale was made then: that merging would cut costs. But it didn't turn out to be true.

The current situation is the 1990s on steroids. And it's made the viability of hospitals and, importantly, the situation for many physicians and other providers much more precarious, much more fragile.

Fragility will lead to cascading failure. In the 1990s, if a hospital failed, chances were that it failed alone. In other words, the physician practices associated with that facility were independent. Certainly, office-based physicians found privileges at another facility. Hospital-based physicians were impacted disproportionately in comparison to their office-based colleagues, but at least there were other hospitals to which to expand their services.

But now, if a hospital, or a merger-bloated hospital system, with its employed or otherwise tightly affiliated physicians, fails, all of those physicians are unemployed. None of them have existing practices independent of the failed hospital.

So, to recap, we have merger for the cure of high costs. And we have a history from the 1990s of a similar trend that resulted in the failure to cut costs culminating in hospital failures. But as opposed to the 1990s, today, many of these merged hospitals not only have traditional hospital-side expenses, they have taken on the huge expenses of employing physicians. Note that it's not just physician labor expense, but the complete expense of operating the practices, from space to equipment to supplies to staff, and so on.

Hospitals are losing the economic bet on employed physicians. So how are hospitals doing with their economic bet on physicians?

A 2014 Kentucky hospital industry study revealed that:

1. The cost to employ a physician in increasing.
2. 58% of hospitals reported annual per-physician losses of more than $100,000 – an increase of 17% over the prior year.
3. Hospitals that hired primary care physicians incurred lower losses on average ($100,000 or less) compared

with hospitalists or specialist physicians (more than $100,000).

4. Specialists also accounted for the greatest losses across the board, representing the only physician provider type to incur more than $200,000 in losses per physician annually.
5. Larger hospital systems faced greater losses, as did larger hospitals. Sixty-six percent of hospitals with more than 200 beds reported losses between $100,000 and $200,000 per provider annually while 33% reported losses greater than $200,000. In smaller hospital systems, and in hospitals with fewer than 200 beds, 88% reported losses less than $200,000, with 66% falling below the $100,000 mark for losses.

Hospitals are losing the bet on integrated delivery networks. And, as to quality, a large study by the National Academy of Social Insurance "found little evidence that integrated delivery networks have reduced costs or improved the quality of care."

Specifically, the study found that:

- Integration of hospitals and physicians results in increased costs.
- Hospital integration into health plan operations and risk-based contracting does not result in shorter lengths of stay or and lower charges per admission.

- Investment in integrated delivery networks leads to a decrease in operating margins and return on capital.

Fragility as a disruptor. This fragility based on business model is a significant internal disruptor, a ticking time bomb.

Keep this fragility in mind as we move along to discuss the other trends attacking the hospital business model from the outside.

Chapter 5
PHYSICIAN-OWNED FACILITIES

Disrupting patient flow to traditional hospitals. The growth of physician-owned facilities, which will increase, is a key disruptor, shifting patient flow out of hospitals.

ASCs. Ambulatory surgery centers, or ASCs as they're commonly known, pull cases, generally the better reimbursed cases, out of the hospital O.R. They offer a significantly cheaper alternative to Medicare, to private payors, and to patients. They also make money for their physician owners.

Currently, there are more than 6,000 ambulatory surgery centers in the United States. There has been a dramatic slowdown in the net addition of ASCs during the last two years. In large part this is due to the fact that hospitals are attempting to remove the competition by purchasing ASCs in the local market.

Notwithstanding that buying spree, it's unlikely that hospitals will be able to stop the shift of cases to the ASC setting.

Certainly, ASCs pull a significant amount of well-reimbursed, commercially covered cases from hospitals. And for many ASCs, depending on the type of case, Medicare reimbursement fits into their business model.

In fact, it's been estimated that, as compared with the cost of care in a hospital setting, ASCs save Medicare and Medicare beneficiaries more than $2.6 billion a year.

The ASC industry estimates that if half of the eligible Medicare cases were shifted from hospital outpatient departments ("HOPDs") to ASCs, there'd be another $2.5 billion in annual savings due to obviating the differential in the amount paid to a hospital for a procedure in an HOPD compared with the amount paid to an ASC for the same procedure.

Payment differential will backfire. Although recent federal budget legislation has reduced some of the benefit of operating as a HOPD, sooner or later the issue of the payment differential will play itself out to disrupt hospitals' futures. HOPD reimbursement will be cut down to ASC levels, leaving hospitals in, at best, a very low profit position or, at worst, a built in loss for each case. In any event, at some point in time, hospitals will be happy to see those cases leave for the ASC setting.

But even if the differential continues to be paid, physicians will continue to invest in and take cases to ASCs and payors will continue to want access to their more cost efficient services.

It's unlikely that hospitals will be able to garner the political support to put up the same roadblocks that they've managed to place on physician-owned hospitals.

Essentially, in order to protect their near monopoly, the investor-owned and non-taxpaying hospitals, many of which are busy employing and otherwise aligning physicians, have claimed that if physicians own hospitals to create teamwork and provide coordinated care, it is bad, but if hospitals own physicians in order to create teamwork and provide coordinated care, it is good. That argument, being nonsensical, will never win in the end.

Even if physicians are prevented from owning hospitals that qualify to treat federal health care program cases, they will continue to invest in smaller hospital facilities focused on private payor cases. They will be able to avoid the low reimbursement that comes from governmental programs and the "no reimbursement" that comes from complete charity care.

Chapter 6
OTHER NEW CLASSES OF COMPETITORS

New sources of disruption. New business models are disrupting the flow of patients, patients who were formerly destined to be referred into a hospital's "world." The growth of physician-owned facilities, which will increase, is a key disruptor, shifting patient flow out of hospitals.

Walk Right In. These models include walk-in clinics of the type opening at retail stores such as Walgreens, RiteAid, and CVS. In fact, CVS, until recently knows as CVS Pharmacy, is now known as CVS Healthcare, which is a clear indication of where they believe healthcare is going.

Other examples are the plethora of walk-in and urgent care facilities built in strip centers and other ease-of-access locations. In fact, in Colorado, Texas, and a number of other states, free-standing emergency rooms, often located near or at intersections close to acute care hospitals, syphon off patients headed to the hospital's O.R. based on their accessibility and their near zero wait times.

The point here is that these types of facilities signal two trends:

First, that non-traditional ventures are disrupting the flow of patients to physicians' offices and to hospital emergency rooms.

Second, and more importantly because this trend has an exponential impact, is the fact that patients don't have the same emotional barriers to obtaining medical care outside of the physician office or hospital setting that they had 20 years ago.

In other words, if care can be obtained in a less intense, less costly, more convenient setting, it's not just insurance carriers who are going to push for it, it's patients who are going to demand it.

Hospitals argue for higher reimbursement for the same services delivered in physicians' offices or at ASCs, and argue against physician-owned hospitals. They portray the issue as the need to protect the bigness of the hospital – the fact that hospitals provide a broad range of care to a broad range of people.

But that's the wrong rationale for today and certainly for tomorrow. Rather, the issue is what should hospitals look like when they are no longer receiving the same influx of patients and are no longer at the center of healthcare delivery.

Despite all of the talk of a "healthcare system" (well, at least by those who have a vested interest in its construction and continuation), that system isn't working the way that hospitals imagined it would, that is, in a hospital-centric way.

The continuation of the hospital-centric system depends on the flow of patients into a catchment system centering around the primary care physicians in the community. Ask any hospital CEO who has spent tens to hundreds of millions of dollars to employ or otherwise align physicians into the hospital's "world," how important they are as the initial feeders into the system.

So, what happens when patients no longer need to see a traditional physician, or a physician at all, to diagnose or treat or to simply assuage someone's healthcare concerns?

Updated house calls. It's 7:00 a.m. on a Wednesday morning and you feel like death warmed over. When you call your doctor's office (not open until 8:30) you know that you'll be told that they might be able to fit you in on Friday.

So, why bother, especially when a physician or nurse practitioner can come see you now. And, at a cost that's probably one-third to one-half what your regular physician charges.

A growing number of services, some telephone request based, some app based, provide or coordinate house call services by physicians, physician assistants and advanced practice nurses.

Telemedicine. If you don't have to see a physician, or even a nurse, in person, why see one? Why not stay at home and simply transmit the same information about your condition to a physician or another provider?

House calls and telemedicine disrupt primary care practices, which will lead to disruption of hospitals. It's not difficult to see that both house call services and telemedicine are disruptive to traditional medical practitioners. In fact, in some states, primary care physicians are exerting pressure on state regulators to make it more difficult for telemedicine and other telehealth companies to operate. Eventually those anticompetitive efforts will fail as patients demand those services – after all, pushing for regulation is the death gasp of any profession or industry; if they can't compete on their own, they turn to the government, and especially to bureaucrats, to protect them.

It requires only slightly more foresight to realize that, in the end, those and other new classes of competitors will not only disrupt traditional office practice, they'll disrupt hospitals as well.

Patients will no longer be following the normal route of (1) go to primary care doctor in an office building on or near a hospital campus; (2) be referred by that physician to a specialist on staff at the same hospital for more detailed diagnosis and care; and (3) receive diagnostic services and treatment at the hospital.

Chapter 7
THE ROLE OF TECHNOLOGY

We're at a technological tipping point. Technology is fuel for the fire of the demise of hospitals as we know them.

We're at a very interesting tipping point in respect to healthcare technology. And, it's not tipping in the hospitals' favor.

For decades, the cost of technology in almost every industry other than healthcare resulted in lower costs to the consumer. But in healthcare, all it did was increase costs.

That history of technology also fed the growth of hospitals. Who, but large facilities, could afford to buy the technology? Wasn't it cheaper and more efficient to, in essence, spread the cost of that technology by locating it in a central location, the hospital, for access by those in the community, both physicians and other providers, as well as by patients?

Thus came the centralizing of technology (read that as medical equipment) from imaging to monitoring to operating rooms themselves.

But today, the cost of technology has shifted. Instead of being more expensive, it is less. In fact, in many cases it's become so much less that it is, or soon will be, affordable at the consumer level, bypassing completely the ASC and physician level.

And, importantly, the size (sometimes there is, effectively, no size at all) of new equipment has shrunk.

Star Trek in the home. Your home. Remember the "tricorder" from Star Trek, the handheld medical diagnostic device? Now, it's time for the real one.

The Qualcomm Tricorder XPRIZE is a $10 million dollar prize for a hand-held tool capable of capturing key health metrics and diagnosing a set of 15 diseases. As of this writing, there are seven finalists.

Tech enables disruption. Technology itself isn't a disruptor; rather, it enables others to disrupt. That includes patients.

It's been estimated that the average waiting time in the U.S. for a doctor's office appointment is over 3 weeks. But how do you know that you need to see a doctor until you see a doctor?

Technology is fast becoming the enabler for devices and for services that permit the disruption of the centuries-old doctor-patient relationship.

Consider the OtoHOME device from Cellscope. It's an iPhone device that allows parents to examine their child's ears and record the result. It then connects them to a doctor for an immediate response.

That's just one example; dozens of other smartphone and wearable devices exist, each of which will reduce visits to traditional primary care doctors. Referrals to specialists (including all of those employed by hospitals) will be reduced, as will diagnostic procedures performed at hospitals.

Tech will also lead to less invasive surgery and to implantable devices that allay more surgery.

It's also bound to lead to the fact that more procedures can be performed in smaller, specialty hospitals and in outpatient settings. Hospitals will no longer need to be everything to everyone. Procedures will move out of general hospitals and into specialty ones. Procedures will move out of hospitals altogether and into ambulatory facilities.

Chapter 8

THE TAKEAWAYS FOR HOSPITALS

1. Hospitals have expanded to become "full service" and have "bought" physicians to capture patients within the hospital system. They claim that by closely aligning physicians they can deliver better care at a lower cost. But they are losing money on employed physicians and there's no evidence that close alignment of physicians results in better care.
2. At the same time, patients are increasingly taking control of their own diagnosis, and in some cases care, via technology.
3. Both technology and new classes of healthcare businesses (e.g., CVS Healthcare, Teladoc, etc.) are enabling patients to bypass traditional brick and mortar facilities (e.g., hospitals and physicians' offices).
4. Patients don't care as much as before whether they see a doctor, a nurse practitioner, or some type of technician. And, for hospitals this is the big one, they don't care as much if they obtain care from someone within the hospital's patient acquisition funnel, or if they get surgery at an ASC or some other non-hospital site. As medicines improve (medicine as the future of surgery) and as

miniaturization permits more procedures outside of the hospital, non-hospital facilities will syphon off a larger and larger percentage of hospital business.

5. Or perhaps patients won't receive care at any facility – perhaps the facility will come to them: Care in a "pod" inside or outside of your house?

Ultimate bottom line: Hospitals will shrink. They will be for the sickest people only. They might become monitoring stations for home care. Many will fail.

Chapter 9

THE TAKEAWAYS FOR PHYSICIANS AND OTHER PROVIDERS

If you think that hospital employment or close alignment is safe, think again.

1. For all physicians and other providers, don't ever be dependent upon a single hospital relationship. In the past, the concern was that that facility might terminate your contract. In the near future, the concern will be that the hospital might not survive.
2. For office-based physicians, and particularly for those in primary care specialties, encourage your patients to adopt new technology and diagnostic tools and offer to be a teacher and participant. Right now, I can hardly get my lab test results from my doctor. When I'm able to get all of my lab tests without her, what makes her think I'll share them with her, specifically? To the extent that she participates in the process, it's far more likely.
3. Freestanding facilities will be the future of facility-based care. If your practice isn't already heavily focused on freestanding facility care, think how you can pivot more in that direction, either now or when you have to. What services can you provide directly to patients, whether

by mobile delivery, in-home delivery, or by way of telemedicine or telehealth?

Ultimate bottom line: Physicians will be impacted by two major thrusts. More and more patient care, including procedures, will move out of the hospital setting into freestanding and other locations, including patients' homes. Technology will enable patients to have their diagnostic information transmitted independent of traditional physicians' offices. Enterprising physicians will see the opportunities in these tectonic shifts. Others will fear them, with good reason.

KNOWLEDGE PRODUCTS

HOW TO PROFIT FROM TELEMEDICINE AND RELATED TECHNOLOGY IN TEXAS

Telemedicine. It's the future and it's arrived no matter what the Medical Board rules or the courts do in any particular case.

Your patients will demand it either way. If not from you, then from someone else.

You can either fear it or you can profit from it. So why not profit from it?

Purchase How to Profit From Telemedicine And Related Technology In Texas now:

Video Version $297 Purchase Now

To purchase **How to Profit From Telemedicine And Related Technology In Texas** go to www.advisorylawgroup.com/knowledgeproducts.html

MEDICAL GROUP MERGERS AND ACQUISITIONS AND ALTERNATIVES

Some days, it seems as if everyone, from anesthesia groups to vascular surgery practices, is talking about selling their practice to a larger group, to private equity investors, or to a hospital.

The reality is that some practices can be sold, some can never be sold, and some have nothing to sell.

The reality also is that there are a number of strategic alternatives to a practice sale.

BREAKING NEWS ON KICKBACKS: THE LATEST ON THE COMPANY MODEL

The recording of Mark F. Weiss' webinar Breaking News On Kickbacks: The Latest On The Company Model. As the healthcare economy becomes more strained, the pace of illegal kickback activity has increased. Join Mark F. Weiss, attorney for the Requestor of OIG Advisory Opinion 13-15, to learn the absolute latest on the so-called Company Model.

Audio Version $279
Video Version $379
Audio and Video Version $379

To purchase **Breaking News On Kickbacks: The Latest On The Company Model** go to
www.advisorylawgroup.com/knowledgeproducts.html

DOUBLE INDEMNITY: PUTTING YOURSELF AT RISK FOR MILLIONS – THE INTERPLAY BETWEEN INSURANCE AND INDEMNIFICATION PROVISIONS IN YOUR HOSPITAL AND PHYSICIAN CONTRACTS

They may look like boilerplate, but your feet might be in the boiler's fire if you haven't properly thought through the impact and interplay of the indemnification and insurance provisions in your contracts with hospitals and with providers.

Audio Version $129
Video Version $179
Video and Audio Versions $179

To purchase **Double Indemnity: Putting Yourself At Risk For Millions – The Interplay Between Insurance And Indemnification Provisions In Your Hospital And Physician Contracts** go to www.advisorylawgroup.com/knowledgeproducts.html

DISRUPTIVE STRATEGIES IN HEALTHCARE: DESIGNING THEM AND DEALING WITH THEM

Believing that the future of the business of healthcare will be a projection of, or incremental improvement over, today's reality is a fool's game.

Although predicting the specifics of the future is impossible, it's certain to involve disruptive strategies. Think, for example, of the disruption to the private practice of medicine resulting from the blossoming hospital-centric worldview. But are you aware of the disruptive strategies aimed at shattering that worldview?

There are only two sides to the healthcare coin: figure out a way to disrupt the current practice model or figure out how to deal with someone else's disruption.

By purchasing you'll understand the role of disruption in healthcare, you'll learn of disruptive events currently on the horizon, you'll learn key elements in designing disruptive strategies and you'll understand how best to protect your practice from someone else's disruption.

Audio Version $107
Video Version $197
Audio and Video Version $197

To purchase **Disruptive Strategies In Healthcare: Designing Them And Dealing With Them** go to www.advisorylawgroup.com/knowledgeproducts.html

THE FAST™ GROUP--MEDICAL GROUP GOVERNANCE FOR TODAY'S MARKET

Does Your Group Suffer From This Governance Defect?

"I'll have to get back to you on that, our board doesn't meet until next Saturday."

In an increasingly competitive, increasingly hospital-centric world, the saying "money likes speed" is more true than ever. Yet many medical groups have doomed themselves to stasis, or worse, as a result of their defective governance structure.

Audio Version $97
Video Version $129
Audio and Video Version $129

To purchase **The Fast™ Group--Medical Group Governance For Today's Market** go to www.advisorylawgroup.com/knowledgeproducts.html

WHY YOUR MEDICAL GROUP NEEDS A NEW CONTRACTING STRATEGY

No matter your political bent, there's no doubt that society is becoming increasingly affected by "we" think, from concepts of shared sacrifice, to paying your fair share, to "giving back."

These notions of community and cooperation present an advantage to local medical groups in fighting off the onslaught of outside competitors.

But that advantage will be lost unless medical groups adopt a contracting strategy that harmonizes with the growing societal trends.

When you watch or listen to this thirty-minute webinar, you'll learn:

- The major general societal trends.
- How those trends impact medical group relationships.
- How those trends impact medical group facility contracting.
- Why having a strategy that ties into those trends.provides you with an essential advantage.

Audio Version $97
Video Version $129
Video and Audio Versions $129

To purchase **Why Your Medical Group Needs A New Contracting Strategy** go to
www.advisorylawgroup.com/knowledgeproducts.html

REVERSE ENGINEERING A NATIONAL TAKEOVER OF YOUR FACILITY CONTRACT

Like a neutron bomb, national or large regional groups wants to take over your facility contract, vaporize your group, and cherry-pick your desirable assets: your physicians and other providers.

By understanding their approach, you'll drastically increase your group's chances for survival.

In the approximately 45 minutes of this recording of an ALG Webinar, you'll learn:

- The strategies and tactics national groups use to approach hospitals.
- What they are saying about you.
- What you can do proactively to inoculate your group against their approach.
- Other tools for protecting your group from planned contractual annihilation.

Audio recording: $397
Complete video of webinar: $497
Audio recording and complete video: $497

To purchase Reverse Engineering A National Takeover Of Your Facility Contract go to
www.advisorylawgroup.com/knowledgeproducts.html

HOW TO DEAL WITH RFPs FOR PHYSICIAN SERVICES

More and more hospitals are disrupting their relationships with hospital-based and office-based physicians.

The favored tool? The request for proposal, commonly known as an "RFP."

How can an RFP be avoided?

Do you respond?

How do you respond?

How can the rules be bent?

These are among the issues discussed in this recording of an ALG Webinar. You'll receive practical and actionable information for your group's immediate application.

After viewing the recording or listening to the audio of this ALG Webinar, you'll have:

- An understanding of the three types of RFPs
- Knowledge of the strategies and tactics used to avoid RFPs
- Awareness of the major defect in the RFP process
- Knowledge of strategies and tactics used to respond to RFPs
- An understanding of the importance of a strategy aimed outside of the RFP process itself

Audio recording $207
Complete video of webinar $297
Audio recording and complete video $297

To purchase **How to Deal With RFPs For Physician Services** go to www.advisorylawgroup.com/knowledgeproducts.html

SPECIAL FREE GIFTS FROM THE AUTHOR

THE IMPENDING DEATH OF HOSPITALS: HOW TO PLAN YOUR PRACTICE'S SURVIVAL FREE WEBINAR RECORDING

You're invited to obtain a free copy of the webinar recording **The Impending Death of Hospitals: How To Plan Your Practice's Survival**, a $297 value.

To obtain your copy, go to
http://www.advisorylawgroup.com/impendinggiveaway.html

SUCCESS OR FAILURE? STRATEGIC TOOLS FOR MEDICAL GROUP LEADERS
FREE BOOK DOWNLOAD

ABOUT THE AUTHOR

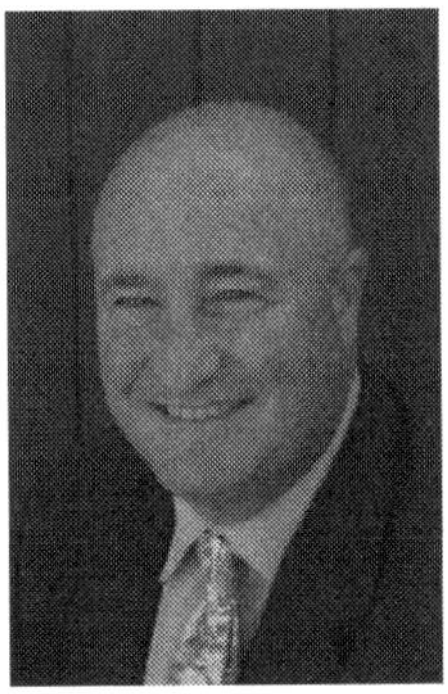

Mark F. Weiss is an expert on the legal and business issues affecting medical groups, entrepreneurial physicians, and healthcare businesses.

Mr. Weiss advises clients nationally on achieving their goals, maximizing their profits and managing their risk of loss.

Lawyers often view the world though a microscope trained to see the minutia of the "legal" issue and, as a result, ignore virtually everything else. As a result, they preach a purely "legal solution" that, quite often, is worthless in terms of any practical benefit for you.

Mr. Weiss views the world differently: He and his firm, The Mark F. Weiss Law Firm, operate on the same entrepreneurial level as do you. He understands that legal issues are intertwined with your business issues and cannot be separated. He understands that psychological and political issues often transcend the obvious issues.

Mr. Weiss is a frequent speaker and the author of more than 200 articles on issues affecting healthcare providers. From 2002 through 2013, he held an appointment as clinical assistant professor of USC's Keck School of Medicine.

Contact Mr. Weiss by phone at 310.843.2800 or email at markweiss@advisorylawgroup.com.

Made in the USA
Monee, IL
19 November 2025

35527299R00039